Nutritional Keys To Your Health

Aries Ford Pemkiewicz

BS, RDN, LDN

Table of contents

DEDICATION

This book is dedicated to GOD for using me as a vessel.

$\mathcal{D}$EDICATION

This book is dedicated to God for using me as a
vessel.
God is worthy of all glory and honor.

ACKNOWLEDGMENTS

To my spiritual leaders, my family and friends who
have supported me through my spiritual walk. I love
you all very dearly and pray abundant blessings over
your lives.

Introduction

You would be very careful of what foods you ingested if you really knew what your body represents and how it can affect your entire life physically and spiritually.

I have counseled people regarding diet and exercise for many years and have realized the measure of great successes appeared when nutrition, health, healing and spiritual well-being were coupled together. Many times nutrition clinicians dive straight into dietary do's and don'ts rather than taking the entire human body and spirit into account. People forget that Jesus walked the earth at one time and knew that it was important to heal body, mind and spirit. Jesus was a fleshly human during that time and experienced many human feelings as we experience today. He grew tired just as we do. This is why he has such compassion for us regarding illnesses and disease. Jesus healed all that requested healing as he walked the earth and taught the gospel. Luke 9:11 says, *"But when the multitudes knew it, they followed him; and he received them and spoke to them about the kingdom of God and healed those who had need of healing."* Keep following Jesus by reading this book because he wants to heal you and get you in shape!

Chapter 1

The Next Feast is on God-eat right and get in shape

Feast - often thought of as a very large, rich, delightfully, well-prepared abundant meal. Everybody gets excited when they hear the word feast. We think "party time!" Why is it that we always look forward to holidays? Is it that we are anticipating spending time with our immediate family and close relatives, or are we just looking forward to the buffet and our own personal "all you can eat contest?" Has anyone thought about a spiritual feast? What is a Godly feast? Jesus spoke about bread from heaven in John Chapter 6:32-35. *"Then Jesus said to them, most assuredly, I say to you, Moses did not give you the bread from heaven, but my Father gives you the true bread from heaven. For the bread of God is he who comes down from heaven and gives life to the world. Then they said to him, Lord, give us this bread always. And Jesus said to them, I am the bread of life. He who comes to me shall never hunger, and he who believes in me shall never thirst."*

John 6:47 says *"Most assuredly, I say to you, he who believes in me has everlasting life."* Not only do you get everlasting life, you also get a chance to develop a relationship with our heavenly Father. God's instructions for his children is to build a relationship with him; a deeper relationship with him. The bible (God in word form) is our food. We can develop a closer relationship with God as we feast on the bible. God wants us to immerse ourselves in him. Now, how can a "Godly Feast" get my body in shape?

Chapter 2

Your Body, God's Temple, Eating Right

Time to get in shape for God's glory! Sometimes we forget that our bodies are precious temples. 1 Corinthians 3:16 says, *"Do you not know that you are the temple of God and that the Spirit of God dwells in you?"* It's important to treat it that way. It's imperative to be healthy. Be careful of what you put into God's Temple. It is true that God has numbered our days on this earth and that he knows us so well that he knows the numbering of the very hairs on our heads. He designed us. He knows our bodies better than we do even though God still allows us to choose how we treat our bodies. He may have planned a long prosperous life for you of many years to teach others of his works, bring others to Christ and to magnify him, but he still allows choices.

Many people suffer from diabetes, hypertension, cancer, obesity and over 25 million people have diabetes. Over 7 million people don't know they have it and over 79 million people have pre-diabetes (which is the medical term given to those who are on the verge of developing diabetes.) 68 million adults have high blood pressure and are taking blood pressure lowering drugs. 71 million people have bad cholesterol levels and more than 35% of the people in the United States are obese.

Health risks are determined by using your weight and height to calculate a number called the body mass index (BMI). BMI under 18.5 = (underweight) and 18.5 - 24.9 = (healthy weight) and 25 - 29.9 = (overweight) and 30 or higher = (obese).

You can also use the waist to hip ratio to determine your risk especially for men with an abundance of muscle that are very active in sports. The BMI chart does not take into account muscle mass. Waist circumference is a good indicator of abdominal fat which is a predictor of risk for obesity related diseases. Overweight and obesity is caused by eating too many calories and inactivity. Health consequences include diabetes, coronary heart disease, cancer, high blood pressure, high lipid levels, stroke, liver and gallbladder disease, sleep apnea, osteoarthritis and gynecological problems. The initial treatment should be dietary changes. In other words, changing what we put in our mouths and how often we bend that elbow.

Health can be defined as the state of complete physical, mental and social well-being or the condition of being sound in body, mind and spirit. Healthy doesn't mean you have to weigh 100 lbs! Healthy can be losing 20 lbs if you are overweight (BMI > 25) or gaining 20 lbs if you are under weight (BMI < 18). I have counseled people and have seen the affects of losing even 10% or gaining 10%. I've seen huge improvements in lab values (blood work) and some people were able to lower their dose of medications or gained the ability to stop their meds with doctor's approval. What kinds of changes do we need to make? Spiritual and physical changes in eating and activity habits. Think about the disciples who followed Jesus. They ate spiritual and physical food. They also exercised with Jesus spiritually and physically. They walked as they were taught. You want to be like the faithful servant. Always ready by sitting at his table and consuming living bread. Allow Jesus to deliver your next meal. Being delivered is going to be our starting point. It's like starting with a clean slate and getting ready for God to lay the foundation. We need to free ourselves and our minds from everything that hinders us from our spiritual and physical goals. I have counseled people for years as a dietitian and have seen the best results with individuals who allowed themselves to let God step in and deliver them from whatever it is that is hindering them from their health goals. Sometimes past mindsets, pain or loneliness can hinder us. One of the biggest hindrances that people express is fear. There are many sources of fear and fear does not come from our heavenly Father. Some forms of fear or other hindrances can come from something that happened during childhood or maybe something was said during your childhood. It can be anything. It can simply be that you had very little to eat and developed a habit of eating everything on your plate when you were served a meal or it could be the feeling of not being loved. Another example can be related to poor education regarding healthy food choices and exercise or just not enough time. Hindrances can be stress related or just pure laziness. Hey, we all get lazy and procrastinate at times. Just know that God can handle whatever it is, but you have to let it go. Even if it is so personal that you may not be able to talk to someone about it, but you can talk to God about it. Psalms 34:4 says, *"I sought the Lord and he heard me, and delivered me from all my fears."* Seek God for deliverance, strength and wisdom. Now that you've recognized it, the rest is easy. Success is waiting for you. Read on and read about how God delivered two other individuals who are now on their way to success.

1. God sent me a woman who was very underweight. She was living at a facility that employed its very own dietitian, but this woman was very persistent with visiting me. Her spouse came along. She struggled for years with anorexia. I understood why she continued to struggle when she and her spouse began to talk. He loved her very much and kept notes on her eating habits and encouraged her daily to increase her food intake. Although he loved her, she felt as if she was being monitored and tightly controlled, which only added to her personal stress and unsuccessfulness. All she needed was for God to deliver her from her personal stress and speak to her husband so that she could gain some control back in her life.

2. I met with a woman of God who loves to read Christian books, but she was still hurting inside. She would eat through her loneliness and stressful days. She wanted to lose weight but couldn't because she had difficulty laying her burdens down. She wasn't going to show up to our appointment, but her husband encouraged her to come to the consultation. She didn't know she was actually meeting God

for some extra encouragement. God doesn't like to see his children in such disarray. He wanted her to know that he would help her to heal and lose the weight she needed to lose to be healthy again. She was taking over 20 medications to alleviate the symptoms of various diseases. She was simply miserable and tired of the way she was feeling. She was tired of people starring at her. God wanted her to know that she was to get up every morning and ask for the spirit of strength to move forward in her weight loss; to ask for the spirit of peace, joy and comfort when she's looking for food to fill the void. During our session, God was able to lift the burdens and heal her heart.

Matthews 11:28-30 says, *"Come to me, all you who labor and are heavy laden, and I will give you rest. Take my yoke upon you and learn from me, for I am gentle and lowly in heart and you will find rest for your souls. For my yoke is easy and my burden is light."*

These were two very different people that were in need of Jesus to take their burdens in order to jump start their health success.

Focus, determination and strength is going to set the foundation of getting our spiritual and physical bodies in shape. We need to be in unity before we go any further. I need you to say out loud Philippians 4:13. *"I can do all things through Christ who strengthens me."* "I am ready to get in shape!" Let's get started! You can do it! You can be a wonderfully beautifully made temple of God, inside and out!

10 quick and easy tips to shape up your food choices

1- Don't drink your calories! Drink water or unsweetened drinks only. Our bodies need at least 6 to 8 glasses of water a day. Water also helps to jump start your metabolism and is required and helps many functions at the cellular level. Sweetened drinks have a quick impact on your blood sugar levels and provide you with lots of empty calories that can cause you to gain weight. A can of soda can have as much calories as a glazed doughnut. Who wants to drink doughnuts when you are trying to lose weight? I've seen people lose 1 to 2 pounds a week just by stopping regular sodas.

2- Don't skip meals! What do we do when we skip a meal? We inhale the entire kitchen table the next time we sit down to eat. This causes us to take in extra calories that will cause weight gain. Instead, try to have a small healthy snack if you are unable to eat within a reasonable time frame.

3- Think balance. Eat a variety of foods at meal time. Don't eat an entire plate of mac-n-cheese for dinner. Be sure to include meat or vegetable protein, starch, vegetables and fruit for dessert. Your body requires a variety of foods to provide vital nutrients to jump start metabolism and initiate other functions at the cellular level.

4- Watch those portions! The plate method is the easiest way to watch portions. No, you cannot pile the plate up like a mountain peak. Half of your plate should be non-starchy vegetables other than beans, corn and potatoes (these are considered starches.) A serving of starch is usually 1/3 to ½ cup serving. You should include 3 oz of meat (which is the size of the palm of your hand) or vegetable protein. Vegetarians are allowed more vegetable proteins or protein substitutes to meet their protein needs. They include beans, nuts, soy, tofu, hummus, peanut butter, almond butter and cheese. A ½ ounce of nuts, 1 tablespoon of peanut butter, ¼ cup of beans or 1 egg is equal to 1 ounce of meat protein. Most people need at least 6 ounces of protein per day. These are general serving guidelines. Please consult a registered dietitian for a personal meal plan and the right serving sizes to meet your individual needs.

5- Balance your carbohydrates (starches such as pasta, rice, bread, beans, potatoes, and corn), fruit, milk and sweets. It's very important that we don't over indulge on these foods. Please contact a registered dietitian or myself if you have diabetes for an individualized meal plan.

6- Watch portions of meat and choose lean meats. 3 oz is a general guideline or the size of the palm of your hand. Choose baked, broiled or grilled meats instead of fried. Watch the cheese. Try adding more vegetable proteins to your meals like peanut butter, nuts and beans instead of meat a few times per week.

7- Eat less fat. Choose lower fat items at restaurants and at the grocery store. Watch servings of salad dressings, butter/margarine, sour cream, cream cheese, cheese, whole milk, and gravies, processed meats (sausage, bacon, and hotdogs.) Choose foods that are baked or grilled. Try rice or almond milk instead of whole milk.

8- Watch the salt. Try not to add salt at the table and reduce processed foods, meats, TV dinners, instant flavored potato/rice boxed mixes and soups. Choose fresh or frozen vegetables most of the time or rinse off the canned vegetables at home.

9- Read food labels and choose lower fat and sodium choices.

10- Try to use other seasonings while cooking instead of salt and butter. Garlic powder, lemon pepper, onion powder and lemon juice are some good substitutions that add flavor. You can also season foods with a variety of vegetables such as colorful peppers and onions.

Weight loss tips for individuals with a BMI over 27
- Eat at least 3 times a day.
- Try not to go more than 5 hrs between meals
- Know when you are hungry. A good rule is a stomach growl.
- Drink a glass of water before each meal and drink water during your meals.
- Don't eat in front of the TV. Your stomach sends the signal to the brain that you are full, but your brain is occupied watching TV which increases your chances of over eating.
- Use smaller plates and bowls.

- Eat slowly and put your fork or spoon down while you chew. Cut your food one bite at a time.
- Brush your teeth after you eat.
- Cook when you are not hungry and drink water while you cook.
- Be careful of emotional eating- Don't eat because you are bored or sad. Read an inspirational book (the bible), call a friend, listen to music or take a walk.

Consult a dietitian for weight gain tips for a BMI < 18 (underweight)

Now we can tackle some of the common road blocks since we have the basic tools to support a generally healthy diet. Road blocks are all the excuses we use and know so well. Which one is yours?

1. I am too stress out.
2. Too exhausted.
3. Not enough time to cook.
4. No time to plan and prepare meals.
5. Everybody else is eating it.
6. I haven't eaten all day.
7. I'm upset.
8. Not sure how to read food lables.
9. No time to exercise.
10. Too expensive to eat healthy and the food taste like cardboard.
11. No exercise equipment.
12. I work at a resturant. How do you expect me to eat healthy?
13. I'm too busy.

14. No one to walk with me, and I don't want to leave the house.
15. I have leg problems.
16. No support.
17. I just went to the salon and my hair is beautiful. I can't exercise now.

Allow me to give you a few simple suggestions, but remember a healthy mind, body and spirit play a part in the chase for God.

1. Exercise helps to relieve stress and so does spiritual meditation. Read the bible. Have you ever encountered someone stressed out and angry reading the bible? The bible is one of the quickest stress relievers that I know.
2. We are only human and we all get tired. We never have a problem finding time to do the pleasurable things that we want to do. Find a time during the day that you aren't so tired to exercise. Find time during the week to shop instead of getting fast processed food.
3. Some days are filled with many errands and work and our families. Try cooking one or two days during the week and freezing leftovers for the other days of the week that you don't have time to cook on. Now you can eat healthy, home cooked meals and you don't have to run out and get fast food.
4. You don't have to eat what everyone else is eating at work or family gatherings. You can make healthy choices and you can choose smaller portions.
5. You don't need special exercise equipment to exercise. You can do chair exercises even if

you have lower body mobility issues. Simply put small water bottles in your hands and raise your arms in an up and down motion. Your body will still get a work out. Your body was designed to move, not just sit around all day. You will feel better once you get moving.

Learn to recognize what affects how much we eat.

1. Going to the movies- rent a movie for home and make air popped corn or limit your portions or avoid snacks at the movies.
2. Watching TV with family- don't eat while watching TV. Chew gum.
3. Employee birthday parties- bring a healthy item and watch portion sizes.
4. Vending machines by my office- bring your own healthy snacks from home.
5. Driving in the car passing fast food- make it a rule never to eat in the car.
6. Going shopping hungry- eat a snack before you go and be careful with coupons. Only buy what you need.
7. Neighborhood parties and pot lucks- bring a healthy dish and eat on a small plate.
8. Your spouse or children are eating high fat-high calorie snacks after dinner- keep healthy low fat snacks in the house for yourself.
9. Buffets- try to avoid these if possible. When going out to eat, please choose healthy options from menus, eat a small healthy snack before

going out and drink plenty of water before and during the meal.

    a. Split entrees
    b. Avoid appetizers and desserts or share
    c. Make healthy substitutions
    d. Watch portions
    e. Be firm and remember your goals

10. I'm having a snack attack!- keep bite size veggies and fruits in sight. Leave all the high fat snack foods on the shelf in the grocery store. Try a handful of nuts and raisins to hold you over until your next scheduled meal time.

Chapter 3

Food Safety and Food Borne Illnesses

Let's protect Gods' Wonderful Temple. Listed are a few Basic Food Safety Precautions to keep you and your family safe from harmful food-borne illnesses, food poisoning and bad bacteria.

- Wash hands, counters and utensils thoroughly.
- Use two separate cutting boards for meats and produce.
- Wash produce thoroughly.
- Disinfect all counter tops before and after food preparation. Especially after raw meats.
- Replace sponges often or wash them in the dishwasher.
- Cook meats until well done.
- Refrigerate food after 2 hours of holding.
- It is best to defrost meats in a sturdy container on the bottom shelf in the fridge instead of on the kitchen counter or sink.
- Always keep cold foods and salads below 40 degrees.
- Good rule of thumb is to keep cold foods cold and hot foods hot!

How do we keep spiritual food safe?

Ask God to protect the seed that was sown in your spirit after you read the bible. Ask him to sow the seeds that you read on good ground and allow it to take root so that you can be blessed just as he speaks of it in Matthew 13:23. *"But he who received seed on the good ground is he who hears the word and understands it, who indeed bears fruit and produces some a hundredfold, some sixty and some thirty. Guard your mind. Meditate on good things."* Philippians 4:8-9 says, *"finally brethren whatever things are noble, whatever things are just, whatever things are pure, whatever things are lovely, whatever things are of good report, if there is any virtue and if there is anything praiseworthy, meditate on these things. The things which you learned and received and heard and saw in me, these do and the God of peace will be with you."*

Basically, protect yourself from negativity and learn how not to receive it. Speak positive words when you encounter people who speak negative words. You need to know what to do around family, friends, co-workers, bosses etc. Look at the book of John to learn the importance of keeping spiritual food safe and your temple clean. Be careful of unclean business taking place in your temple. Jesus cleaned out the temple and told them not to make his father's house a mess of uncleanliness. Uncleanliness can be in the form of ungodly behavior and or harmful ways of treating our bodies. The people couldn't understand Jesus when he told them that he would destroy the temple and raise it up in 3 days. They thought to themselves how can someone tear down a temple and then rebuild it in 3 days when it had taken 46 years to build. Jesus was actually talking about his temple, which was within him. Many people have experienced poor eating and activity habits for years and feel as if it's going to be very difficult to change. It's not impossible with Jesus. It is very important for

Jesus to protect the temple of God both spiritually and physically. Jesus spoke of both physical and spiritual temples.

In the book of John, Jesus died for our sins and was raised up in 3 days. His temple is now our temple as we abide in him. His temple was his body when he was man. His spirit is now able to live within us, if we allow him. He wants to come in, but it is important that we protect our temples and keep it clean. Protect your temple with prayer and clean thoughts by keeping the commandments and striving to live righteously. Ephesians 5:10 says,*" finding out what is acceptable to the Lord and have no fellowship with the unfruitful works of darkness, but rather expose them."*

Think of food safety becoming temple safety. Do not ingest anything that is going to harm your temple, such as worldly thoughts or worldly things. Let your mind meditate on the goodness of God and only let your conduct be worthy of the gospel of Christ. Continue to consume good healthy food; food from our heavenly Father which allows us to continue to grow and stay connected with God. Jesus speaks about the true vine in John 15. Jesus says that if we abide in him then he can abide in us (our temple.) We have the ability to bear much fruit; to bear the goodness of God. Ephesians 5:8 says, *"The fruit of the spirit is in all goodness, righteousness and truth."*

If we abide in Jesus we can grow this fruit, but without him we can do nothing. We have the ability to grow spiritually and help others to grow spiritually and God will be glorified. We are no longer in darkness once we have accepted Jesus. The light of the Lord is now within us. Jesus is the light. We can ask what we desire from God when we allow Jesus to abide in our temples. Continue to abide in Jesus by reading the word of God and having faith. Allow him to dwell in your heart, provide you with strength and unspeakable love from God.

I think Apostle Paul says it best in Ephesians 3:14-20. *"For this reason I bow my knees to the Father our Lord Jesus Christ, from whom the whole family in heaven and earth is named, that he would grant you according to the riches of his glory to be strengthened with might through his spirit in the inner man, that Christ may dwell in your hearts through faith, that you being rooted and grounded in love, may be able to comprehend with all the saints what is the width and length and depth and height to know the love of Christ which passes knowledge , that you may be filled with all the fullness of God. Now to him who is able to do exceedingly abundantly above all that we ask or think, according to the power that works in us to him be glory in the church by Christ Jesus to all generations forever and ever. Amen."*

Chapter 4

Let's Go Shopping!

<u>Grocery shopping tips</u>

- Make a list to save time and money. It only makes sense to look at the sales paper to determine what's on sale first. Look in your cabinets and see what you really need from the sale items to start making healthy meals at home. Now you are ready to create a list to provide meals for the next 7 days or so. Consider vegetarian meals during the week as well.

- Start in the produce aisle first. Look for colorful, nutrient rich fruits and vegetables. Bright colors indicate more antioxidants which help to protect the body. Produce is also rich in fiber and very low in calories. Half of your lunch and dinner plate should be filled with selections from the produce aisle.

- Next we can look for dry items and save the cold items for last. We need to keep those items cold as long as possible.

- Shop for whole grain items such as breads, pasta, and rice. Don't forget the nuts and beans.

Now we can shop for lean skinless meats, fish and low fat and fat free dairy. You can also replace your dairy with rice or almond milk and green leafy vegetables. Lean meats include skinless chicken and turkey breast, beef cuts without marbling (fat), (sparingly) round steak tenderloin, sirloin tips and center cuts. Don't forget to keep raw meats on the bottom of the cart to prevent cross contamination.

Frozen items should be last in order to keep them frozen as long as possible during travel. You can shop for frozen unbreaded meats/fish, fruits, vegetables, whole grain breakfast items and sorbets. Sometimes frozen foods can be more cost effective, and they are packed with nutrients.

Try not to shop for foods that have a lot of added ingredients such as fat, sugar and salt such as : processed foods, boxed rice, pasta and potato mixes, canned soups, TV dinners, breaded meats and vegetables, bacon, sausage, tuna canned in oil, beans cooked in lard, vegetables cooked in cream or cheese sauces, fried vegetables, sweet rolls, doughnuts, pastries, biscuits, fried tortillas, sugar coated cereals, juices or drinks sweetened with sugar, fruit canned in heavy syrup, 2% or whole milk, regular cheese, yogurt with sugar, hot dogs, and meat with skin.

These foods are high in calories, fat, sodium and or sugar. Moderation is the key as well as finding these choices with reduced sodium, sugar and fat. Canned foods tend to be high in sodium. Try to purchase reduced sodium or no added salt. You can also rinse your vegetables thoroughly to remove the sodium before consuming. Purchase snacks that are low in fat, sodium, sugar and free of trans fats or hydrogenated oils. Good snacks include bite size raw fruits and vegetables, unsalted pretzels, animal crackers, Jello or pudding. Sherbet and sorbet are good choices. Good snack choices include items that contain less than 5 grams of fat per serving.

You never know what you might get when you go shopping with the Lord. There are a variety of different foods mentioned in the bible. After reading about several food items, God showed me how some of these foods were connected to certain individuals in certain situations. Many individuals are in need of something from God. There are many bible verses that correlate food in situations to show great favor and blessings from God. As you read scriptures, God will began to show you the relationship of the individuals and what they ingested during or while God gave them favor, gifts and the desires of their hearts. There are also times where God speaks of foods to certain people to assure them that favor was coming their way or would come their way through their obedience.

Some of my favorite shoppers in the bible include Moses, Aaron and the children of Israel. What did they put in their grocery basket? The list included milk, honey, bread, almonds, olives, pomegranates, vines, water, wheat and barley. Some foods represent spiritual goodness, knowledge, power, delightfulness, love and truth. Let's shop for milk and honey. It is the land of goodness, the land of richness, the sweet land that everyone longs for because it lacks nothing. It's the place in your life where blessings will overtake you. God promises us earthly blessings as well as eternal life in heaven. This land for us can be many things that we desire. It can be the financial blessing that we've been waiting for, a home, a car, success, a major breakthrough, healing physically or mentally, relationship reconnections, a greater connection to God for you and your family or any other desires of your heart. The children of Israel were held captive in Egypt and prayed for God to deliver them. God sent Moses, Aaron and then Joshua to lead them through the wilderness to the promise land, the land of milk and honey.

They suffered along the way just as we do when we are going through trials in life. They complained along the way. Sounds like us when we are going through tough times in life. Our trials are how we go through the wilderness. Sometimes we have to endure and go through the wilderness in order to obtain God's promise of abundant blessings. God still provided for them and took care of them as they were going through the wilderness. God was able to teach the children of Israel through Moses about his power through miracles signs, and wonders.

Sometimes God has to show you something in order for you to believe and be encouraged. God taught about his commandments and his laws as well as reviewed them in Deuteronomy because they are of such importance. God was molding and shaping just as he has to mold and shape us in order to get us ready to enter the land of milk and honey. God needs to know for sure that you will listen to him, be obedient and not forget him after he brings you out of your trial. Deuteronomy 8:2-3 says, *"And you shall remember that the Lord your God led you all the way these forty years in the wilderness to humble you and test you, to know what was in your heart, whether you would keep his commandments or not. So he humbled you, allowed you to hunger and fed you with manna which you did not know nor did your father know, that he might make you know that man shall not live by bread alone, but man lives by every word that proceeds from the mouth of the Lord."*

You must continue to live by the word of the Lord and always make him priority. God says this next in Deuteronomy 8:11-18, *"beware that you do not forget the Lord your God by not keeping his commandments, his judgments and his statues which I command you today, lest when you have eaten and are full and have built beautiful houses and dwell in them and when your herds and flocks multiply and your silver and your gold are multiplied and you forget the Lord your God who brought you out of the land of Egypt from the house of bondage who led you through that great and terrible wilderness in which were fiery serpents and scorpions and thirsty land where there was no water, who brought water for you out of the flinty rock, who fed you in the wilderness with manna, which your fathers did not know, that he might humble you and that he might test you to do you good in the end, then you say in your heart, my power and the might of my hand have gained me this wealth and you shall remember the Lord your God, for it is he who gives you power to get wealth that he may establish his covenant which he swore to your fathers as it is this day."*

Don't forget God after he brings you out of your trials, after he gives you a supernatural blessing according to your hearts desires, after he allows you to obtain a new job or career, after he goes before you and fights your battles, after he provides you with finances or showers you with love, joy, strength, peace, freedom, wisdom, healing, comfort and good health. Continue to give him all the glory and thank him for all that he has done in your life. Continue to strive to fulfill your purpose in him. Continue to obey his voice and lead others to Jesus. Continue to walk in love and forgive others. Continue to remain humble. We are all in this together. Deuteronomy 6:4-5 says, *"Hear, O Israel: the Lord our God is one! You shall love the Lord your God with all your heart, with all your soul and with all your strength."* Deuteronomy 7:9 says, *"therefore know that the Lord your God, he is God, the faithful God who keeps covenant and mercy for a thousand generations with those who love him and keep his commandments."* Deuteronomy 7:13 says, *"And he will love you and bless you and multiply you, he will also bless the fruit of your womb and the fruit of your land, your grain and your new wine and oil, the increase of your cattle and the offspring of your flock in the land of which he swore to your fathers to give you."* God wants to bless you and everything around you and give you eternal life. Nothing gets better than that. Be obedient and remain humble. The land of milk and honey is yours! That's what I'm going for!

Chapter 5

The Perfect Food Label

Have you ever thought of a food label being a special instruction from God? Isaiah 28:23, 26, 29 says, "*Give ear and hear my voice, listen and hear my speech. For he instructs him in right judgment, his God teaches him.*" This also comes from the Lord of hosts, who is wonderful in counsel and excellent in guidance. Reading the biblical food label (the bible) is very important for guidance. God is able to teach us the right judgments and guide us through life towards eternal life. All we have to do is read it. The bible is life, light and the word in paper form. The word is the spirit of God. This is one of the ways the Lord speaks to you. You are actually reading him. It's not just a bible. He's standing in front of you. This label is his garment. He wears a garment of words for conversation; a garment of words for wisdom, a garment of words for comfort, love, strength, and joy. And a garment that is a provider and a protector; a garment that fights battles. Basically a garment that can and will meet our every need if we allow him to. A garment that connects us to him. God will move and connect with you via revelations as you read the bible. His revelations are teaching lessons guided by the Holy Spirit that no man can teach. He is the perfect label! Every ingredient has already been planned and included to make the perfect meal. The portions are just right and the meal is guaranteed to taste good!

Reading product food labels are important, too. God also guides us through those as well regarding our physical health. Reading labels is another form of the wisdom that God has just gifted you with. There are two types of label reading. What to look at when you have time and what to look at when you don't have much time such as during grocery shopping.

Look for these basic label readings at a glance while shopping. Fat and sodium content is the most important items to read on the food label during shopping if you are new at reading labels and want to save time. You can worry about the serving size and carbohydrate count when you get home. Items high in fat will most likely be high in calories. Eating too much fat makes us fat. Healthy eating means reducing the fat and sodium we consume. You also want to be familiar with high fiber choices. Choose food items with greater than 5 grams of fiber per serving.

Don't forget that it is also important to know what's in your food. Let me show you what to look for on a label. Find a label in your kitchen and follow along with me.

Serving size- determines the amount of calories and nutrients in one serving. You have to add more calories if you decide to eat more or the entire package. The same idea goes for fat, sodium and carbohydrates as well.

Fat grams- Compare products and choose foods with the least amount of total fat grams- less than 5 grams of fat per serving for snack foods.

Sodium- Try to choose foods lowest in sodium. 140mg is a good goal per serving.

Carbohydrates- One serving of carbohydrates is equivalent to 15 grams of carbohydrates. A sugar gram is just a component of carbohydrates. Carbohydrates break down into sugar. Seek a dietitian if you want a personalized carbohydrate controlled meal plan.

Fiber- Try to choose items with 5 grams or more per serving.

Chapter 6

Keep Moving and Watch GOD Move

There are many benefits to physical activity. Dancing to your favorite song like nobody's watching can jump start your weight loss, maintain your weight and prevent further weight gain. Other benefits include:

- Preventing and managing health conditions and disease, strengthen bones to reduce falls, improves heart health, and improves blood sugar and blood pressure levels as well.
- Boost energy levels by delivering more oxygen to your tissues.
- Improves your mood, releases stress and improves confidence. You look better and feel better about yourself.
- Promotes better sleep at night.

Consider at least 30 minutes of daily physical activity. You may need to increase your minutes if your goal is weight loss. Exercising large muscle groups is an effective way to burn fat and gain muscle. Add weight baring exercises to your weekly workouts. One pound weight loss per week is equivalent to burning 3500 calories. That's 500 calories a day or a 16 oz. soda and 3 small cookies per day. You can start slow and build up to 30-60 minutes a day. Some people do 10 minutes three times a day initially. Do what works

34

for you. Stop when you feel abnormally tired and stay hydrated by drinking plenty of water. It is suggested to consult with your physician if you are just starting with exercise for your own safety.

10 Tips to increase your physical activity

1. Post a reminder on the fridge, on the TV and on the bathroom mirror.

2. Put the exercise equipment in front of the TV.

3. Keep your gym shoes in the car or by the front door.

4. Leave an exercise DVD on the coffee table.

5. Hang an activity calendar up at work.

6. Walk on your lunch break.

7. Make a walking date with a friend.

8. Power-walk listening to bible verses.

9. Take the stairs.

10. Park far and walk.

Exercise is vital just as being on the move for God is vital. Do you want to see God move on your behalf? You need to move if you want to see God move. In other words, you will see more blessings manifest in your life as you move towards telling people about his greatness (the mighty works of his hands) Psalms 105. Encourage those who may be lost to accept Jesus as their Lord and Savior. Romans10:9-10 says, *"That if you confess with your mouth the Lord Jesus and believe in your heart that God has raised him from the dead, you will be saved. For the heart one believes to righteousness and with the mouth confession is made to salvation."* Be on the move by reading your bible more. Work that brain, hand and optical muscle by turning the pages and reading! The more you grow in the word, the more you will see God move on your behalf. The more miracles you will see happen in your life. You will see God move more in your life when you allow God to move in your life by sowing seeds of his word into your spirit. Get on the move!

Chapter 7

Wear the Right Clothes

Comfortable, good fitting clothing and shoes are important before exercising. God has clothes for you too; spiritual clothing. It's called spiritual armor and it's what we all need before we step out the door. Not putting your spiritual clothes on is like leaving the house to exercise at the gym without anything on your feet. Really, who does that? Putting on the armor of God is a part of the preparation of the spiritual fight. It's how God prepares you as he fights your battles. He's walking with you every day as your leave the door of your home, but you need to be suited up. It's for your own protection.

Don't forget to put on the armor. Ephesians 6:13-18 says," *Therefore take up the whole armor of God that you may be able to withstand in the evil day and having done all to stand. Stand therefore, having girded your waist with truth, having put on the breastplate of righteousness and having shod your feet with the preparation of the gospel of peace, above all, taking the shield of faith with which you will be able to quench all the fiery darts of the wicked one and take the helmet of salvation and the sword of the spirit, which is the word of God, praying always with all prayers and supplication in the spirit, being watchful to this end with all perseverance and supplication for all the saints.*" Don't forget to speak boldly about the mighty works of the Lord.

Chapter 8

Staying Motivated!

Staying motivated during exercising and eating healthy becomes easier when you don't forget to recognize when you are doing well. Self-monitor, seek support, and add variety to your routines. Keep track of your weight and eating habits with a food record and activity record. If you stumble, that's ok, just get back up and keep trying. Set goals and reward yourself with non-food related activities. One of my friends said she was going to start exercising with Jesus every day. Jesus would come to her door and they would go walking together. One day it was 95 degrees out. She took one step outside and said, "Jesus, you'll have to meet me tomorrow." It's ok to take a break for a day or two. It's just important not to stop.

The same thought applies to the bible or attending church. You may miss a few days or even a week. Just remember to get back on track. Do you ever wonder how the disciples stayed motivated? They learned how to depend on God through Jesus. Luke 9:16 says, *"Then Jesus took the five loaves and the two fish and looking up to heaven; he blessed and broke them and gave them to the disciples to set before the multitude."* The disciples watched Jesus pray to God to stretch the five loaves enough to feed thousands of people. Not only did the power of God motivate the disciples, but it also motivated the people to keep following Jesus. They continued to follow Jesus because they knew they would not only get a meal, but also be healed and whatever else they were seeking. We would do the same. Sometimes we go to a company party, barbeque or a seminar because we know there's going to be food there. Everybody likes to eat. Listen, Jesus can keep you motivated and encouraged just as he kept the disciples motivated and encouraged. Look at Mark 8:17. *"And Jesus being aware of it said to them why do you reason because you have no bread? Do you not yet perceive nor understand? Is your heart still hardened?"* Basically, Jesus said "don't you know who I am and what I can do through my Father?" They walked with Jesus and saw all the miracles and still needed encouragement at times.

Jesus has done so much in our lives and we still doubt the power of God. We doubt that God can repair any situation. We doubt that God can help us toward our weight goals. We forget to ask him to help us with our diet and weight management just as we forget to ask him to help us in other areas of our lives. Maybe you fall into the category of not forgetting to ask him for help in areas of your life, but how is your faith? You can't ask without having faith and walking in it. Feeding our spirit with God's word gives us power and wisdom. God's word signifies life in every situation we are faced with or going to face. His word gives us the power to overcome life's' hurdles. What's so hard about reading a verse 3 times a day? We eat three times a day and some of us eat more than that.

Intertwine physical and spiritual food for the Glory of God. While you feed your physical body, keep in mind to eat spiritual food for God's glory. A verse with each meal and snack should get you through the bible at the speed of light and guaranteed to get you closer to our heavenly Father. Let him motivate you!

Have you ever thought about how food can allow you to be in right standing with God? Take a walk with me through the New and the Old Testament.

Chapter 9

Bread

Oh, how we love bread. We cannot live by bread alone, but we must live by every word that proceeds from the mouth of the Lord (Deuteronomy 8:3). Well, unleavened bread in exodus was to be consumed as God directed and God gave further instructions in Leviticus as well. It was a sacrificial offering directed by God to remind us of his mercy and goodness. It was also a form of protection. Now we have living bread called Jesus! Consuming the bread of Jesus will provide us a direct connection to God.

John chapter 6:32-35 say *"Then Jesus said to them, most assuredly, I say to you, Moses did not give you the bread from heaven, but my Father gives you the true bread from heaven. For the bread of God is he who comes down from heaven and gives life to the world. Then they said to him, Lord, give us this bread always. And Jesus said to them, I am the bread of life. He who comes to me shall never hunger, and he who believes in me shall never thirst."* In Exodus, God rained bread from heaven as a test after the children of Israel complained. Today, Jesus is our test. Will you accept Jesus as your Lord and personal Savior? Hint: pass the test and say yes.

Chapter 10

Water

Drinking water is vital in order for the human body to survive. Living water is also vital in order for us to remain in right standing with God. Jesus sent the Holy Spirit to help us through. John 16:7-11 says, *"Nevertheless I tell you the truth. It is to your advantage that I go away, for if I do not go away, the helper will not come to you, but if I depart, I will send him to you. And when he comes, he will convict the world of sin, and of righteousness and of judgment, of sin because they do not believe in me, of righteousness, because I go to my Father and you see me no more, of judgment, because the ruler of this world is judged."*

The Holy Spirit is here to help us live righteously. That's the small voice that we hear when we may not be making the right decisions or the feelings we get when we are making the right decisions. The Holy Spirit guides and teaches us. John 14:25-26 says, *"These things I have spoken to you while being present with you but the helper, the Holy Spirit whom the Father will send in my name, he will teach you all things and bring to your remembrance all things that I said to you."*

The Holy Spirit is vital living water. You cannot enter the kingdom without it. John 3:5-7 says, *"Jesus answered; most assuredly, I say to you, unless one is born of water and the Spirit, he cannot enter the kingdom of God. That is born of flesh is flesh, and that which is born of the Spirit is spirit. Do not marvel that I said to you, you must be born again."* The Holy Spirit is a requirement to enter the kingdom and it is needed to cleanse us as well.

Ephesians 5:27 says, *"That he might sanctify and cleanse her with the washing of water by the word, that he might present her to himself a glorious church, not having spot or wrinkle or any such thing, but that she should be holy and without blemish."*

Water by the word cleanses your temple from the inside out. Don't forget to drink your water.

Chapter 11

Spices and Oils

Have you ever cooked with or used myrrh, cinnamon, cane, cassia, stact, onycha, galbanum, spikenard, frankincense or olive oil? These are spices and oils with spiritual significance. Some of these served as special ingredients for sweet smelling incense used during sacrificial offerings in the Old Testament and some are used in anointing oils. Today, we are the perfume and incense during worship, praise and prayer. We must offer sweet smelling acceptable worship and prayer. Psalm 141:2 says,"*Let my prayer be set before you as incense, the lifting up of my hands as the evening sacrifice.*"

John 4:23-24 says, *"but the hour is coming, and now is when the true worshippers will worship the Father in spirit and truth for the Father is seeking such to worship him. God is spirit and those who worship him must worship in spirit and truth."* Give God your best spices if you really desire something from God. Don't forget to add the oil. Jesus was anointed throughout the bible with precious perfumed oils. Matthew 26:7 says," *a woman came to him having an alabaster flask of very costly fragrant oil, and she poured it on his head as he sat at the table"* and again in John 12:3 it says, *"Then Mary took a pound of very costly oil of spikenard, anointed the feet of Jesus and wiped his feet with her hair."* Anoint yourself with oil before prayer as stated in Matthew Chapter 6 and Psalm 23. Don't forget to include your family and your home as well.

Chapter 12

Fruit

Good fruit is nutritious, sweet and juicy. Bearing good fruit is another way to grow your relationship with God. John 15:1-2 says, *"I am the true vine, and my Father is the vinedresser. Every branch in me that does not bear fruit he takes away and every branch that bears fruit he prunes, that it may bear more fruit."* Jesus is telling us that you have to go through him to connect to God and you will be trimmed if you don't bear good fruit, but the good news is that you are enabled to increase good fruit of the spirit if you share what you have and have the desire to grow. An example of fruit is your behavior. People are always watching what you do even when you don't think they are watching you. You want to exhibit behavior that gives God glory and behavior that will please God. You will continue to see an increase in spiritual growth as you pray and teach others about God.

Now you are probably wondering what exhibits bad fruit. Look at Matthew 7:15-20. *"Beware of false prophets who come to you in sheep's clothing, but inwardly they are ravenous wolves. You will know them by their fruits. Do men gather grapes from thorn bushes or figs from thistles? Even so, every good tree bears good fruit, but a bad tree bears bad fruit. A good tree cannot bear bad fruit, nor can a bad tree bear good fruit. Every tree that does not bear good fruit is cut down and thrown into the fire. Therefore by their fruits you will know them."*

Also, take special note of what is spoken of in Ephesians 5:10. *"Finding out what is acceptable to the Lord and have no fellowship with the unfruitful works of darkness, but rather expose them."* Some people will smile in your face and talk about you behind your back. Some people will smile in your face, but look the other way when you've lost a job or suffered an illness. It's not difficult to know the difference between good and bad fruit. It's all about loving instead of judging those who are in need as well as making sure your behavior pleases God and connects others to God. Don't be the one who continues to bear bad fruit or practice lawlessness and lose connection and have the Lord speak as stated in Matthew 7:23. *"And then I will declare to them, I never knew you, depart from me, you who practice lawlessness!"* Make sure that you know that you know that God knows you. Bear good fruit and lots of it!

Chapter 13

Meat and Salt

Burnt offerings were to be without blemish. There were times that God requested that these offerings be seasoned with salt. In other words, God wants your best. We are free from sacrificing animals because Jesus died for us and was the ultimate blood sacrifice. We are covered under the blood of Jesus. Today we can ask for forgiveness, give thanks, gratitude and appreciation by sacrificing our meat intake during a spiritual fast. Our bodies are expected to be a living sacrifice for God. Jesus teaches believers about being the salt of the earth. Matthew 5:13,16 says, *"You are the salt of the earth; but if the salt loses its flavor, how shall it be seasoned? It is then good for nothing but to be thrown out and trampled underfoot by men. Let your light shine before men, that they may see your good works and glorify your Father in Heaven."*

Salt adds flavor and it's a parable for letting people see God's goodness through you. Jesus also speaks about walking in peace in Mark 9:49. *"For everyone will be seasoned with fire and every sacrifice will be seasoned with salt. Salt is good, but if the salt loses its flavor, how will you season it? Have salt in yourselves, and have peace with one another."* You see, we are the spiritual salt of sacrifice. We must practice peace and love as direct instructions from God. Continue to offer your best by abiding in Jesus and fleeing from sin. You don't want to miss out on the kingdom of heaven. Live by faith and strive to have a personal relationship with God. Request to

47

know him a way that no one knows him. There are so many people sitting in church or at home today that think they know God, but they have only scratched the surface. An increase in a personal relationship is when your faith begins to grow beyond measure because God just performed something supernatural in your life; something that no human being could ever do. Just think about it for a minute. If you can't think of anything just ask him to do something for you, but remember it will require you to do something as well. Don't forget the other spices to add to your sacrifice.

Our temple is a living sacrifice. It is an expectation from God that we strive to live holy and acceptable. You have all the ingredients. There is no excuse. Try to be the best that you can be and give God all glory.

Chapter 14

Are You There?

Have you been seeking a connection or reconnection to God? Maybe you or you may know someone who feels like the prodigal son. You feel unworthy and like you have sinned against your family and/or our heavenly Father. Maybe you thought, said or imagined something ungodly. Today is your day to get it right with God. Luke 15:7 says, "*I say to you that likewise there will be more joy in heaven over one sinner who repents than over ninety-nine (99) just persons who need no repentance.*" You are not alone. Repent and the angles in heaven will cheer and dance for you.

The book of Romans says in 3:23 *"for all have sinned and fall short of the glory of God, being justified freely by his grace through the redemption that is in Christ Jesus, whom God set forth as a propitiation by his blood, through faith to demonstrate his righteousness, because in his forbearance God had passed over the sins that were previously committed to demonstrate at the present time his righteousness, that he might be just and the justifier of the one who has faith in Jesus."* Romans 8:2 says, *"For the law of the spirit of life in Christ Jesus has made me free from the law of sin and death."*

Accept Jesus into your life. Romans 10:9-10 says, *"That if you confess with your mouth the Lord Jesus and believe in your heart that God has raised him from the dead, you will be saved. For the heart one believes to righteousness and with the mouth confession is made to salvation."* Find a church and get baptized in the name of the Father and of the Son and of the Holy Spirit. Seek spiritual growth and become a living sacrifice to God. Romans 12:1-2 says, *"I beseech you therefore brethren, by the mercies of God, that you present your bodies a living sacrifice, holy, acceptable to God, which is your reasonable service. And do not be conformed to this world, but be transformed by the renewing of your mind, that you may prove what is that good and acceptable and perfect will of God."*

Ask God to guide you and keep you acceptable. God renews our mind by his words. Reading his words is a daily mind renewal and it will help to guide you and keep you on the right path. Increase your faith. Romans 10:17 says, *"So then faith comes by hearing and hearing by the word of God."* Your faith will be increased by reading about the word of God, listening for God to speak to you and learning more about God through good spiritual leaders that God has imparted into. Your faith will continue to grow as God teaches you how to recognize his blessings and revelations for you to impart into others. Serve God with all you have through prayer, praise and worship, thankfulness, walking in love and speaking to others about the mighty works of his hands! There's always a way and an opportunity to tell others about God in everything we do. Many times people are thirsting for an opportunity to talk or hear about the goodness of the Lord but are afraid to say anything. Just try it and watch how God begins to work in your life and the other person's life. Speaking of his goodness brings joy, healing and many other blessings that God knows his children need. Again, serve God with all you got! It is the best way to get your body, mind and spirit in shape!

ABOUT THE AUTHOR

Please visit my website at
www.AriesFord.org

For nutrition consults and many other inspirational reading materials.

You may have seen appearances

by Aries on WXII 12

"Parents balancing work and family",

"Moms saving Time",

TCP and Triad Fitness and Health Magazines

www.ingramcontent.com/pod-product-compliance
Lightning Source LLC
Chambersburg PA
CBHW070338290526
45791CB00003B/1376